DASH DIET

A step to step guide on dash diet with low sodium recipes to lower your blood pressure

Dr Rowan Theo

Table of Contents

CHAPTER ONE

Dash diet
The Complete Beginner's Guide to the DASH Diet

High blood stress impacts extra than a thousand million human beings worldwide — and that wide variety is rising.

In truth, the wide variety of human beings with excessive blood stress has doubled in the remaining forty years — a extreme fitness concern, as excessive blood stress is related to a better hazard of situations together with coronary heart sickness, kidney failure and stroke.

As food plan is idea to play a chief function in the improvement of excessive blood stress, scientists and policymakers have engineered precise nutritional techniques to assist lessen it.

This article examines the DASH food plan, which become designed to fight excessive blood stress and decrease human beings's hazard of coronary heart sickness.

What Is the DASH Diet?

Dietary Approaches to Stop Hypertension, or DASH, is a food plan advocated for those who need to save you or deal with hypertension — additionally called excessive blood stress — and decrease their hazard of coronary heart sickness.

The DASH food plan makes a specialty of end result, greens, complete grains and lean meats.

The food plan become created after researchers observed that excessive blood stress become lots much less common in those who observed a plant-primarily based totally food plan, together with vegans and vegetarians.

That's why the DASH food plan emphasizes end result and greens at the same time as containing a few lean protein reassets like bird, fish and beans. The food plan is low in pork, salt, brought sugars and fats.

Scientists consider that one of the fundamental motives human beings with excessive blood stress can advantage from this food plan is as it reduces salt consumption.

The normal DASH food plan software encourages no extra than 1 teaspoon (2,three hundred mg) of sodium consistent with day, that is in step with maximum countrywide recommendations.

The decrease-salt model recommends no extra than

three/four teaspoon (1,500 mg) of sodium consistent with day.

SUMMARY

The DASH food plan become designed to lessen excessive blood stress. While wealthy in end result, greens and lean proteins, it restricts pork, salt, brought sugars and fats.

Potential Benefits

Beyond decreasing blood stress, the DASH food plan gives some of capacity advantages, such as weight reduction and decreased most cancers hazard.

However, you shouldn't assume DASH that will help you drop some pounds on its own — because it become designed essentially to decrease blood stress. Weight loss may also absolutely be an brought perk.

The food plan influences your frame in numerous ways.

Lowers Blood Pressure

Blood stress is a degree of the pressure placed on your blood vessels and organs as your blood passes via them. It's counted in numbers:

- Systolic stress: The stress on your blood vessels whilst your coronary heart beats.

- Diastolic stress: The stress on your blood vessels among heartbeats, whilst your coronary heart is at rest.

Normal blood stress for adults is a systolic stress under a hundred and twenty mmHg and a diastolic stress under eighty mmHg. This is commonly written with the systolic blood stress above the diastolic stress, like this: a hundred and twenty/eighty.

People with a blood stress analyzing of 140/ninety are taken into consideration to have excessive blood stress.

Interestingly, the DASH food plan demonstrably lowers blood stress in each wholesome human beings and people with excessive blood stress.

In research, human beings at the DASH food plan nonetheless skilled decrease blood stress although they didn't shed pounds or limit salt consumption.

However, whilst sodium consumption become restricted, the DASH food plan diminished blood stress even further. In truth, the best discounts in blood stress had been visible in human beings with the bottom salt consumption.

These low-salt DASH food plan effects had been maximum staggering in those who already had excessive blood stress, decreasing systolic blood stress via way of means of a median of 12 mmHg and diastolic blood stress via way of means of five mmHg.

In human beings with everyday blood stress, it decreased systolic blood stress via way of means of four mmHg and diastolic via way of means of 2 mmHg.

This is in step with different research which screen that

proscribing salt consumption can lessen blood stress — specifically in the ones who've excessive blood stress.

Keep in thoughts that a lower in blood stress does now no longer continually translate to a reduced hazard of coronary heart sickness.

CHAPTER TWO

May Aid Weight Loss

You will in all likelihood revel in decrease blood stress at the DASH food plan whether or not or now no longer you shed pounds.

However, in case you have already got excessive blood stress, probabilities are you've got been cautioned to shed pounds.

This is due to the fact the extra you weigh, the better your blood stress is in all likelihood to be.

Additionally, dropping weight has been proven to decrease blood stress.

Some research endorse that human beings can shed pounds at the DASH food plan.

However, the ones who've misplaced weight at the DASH food plan had been in a managed calorie deficit — which means they had been instructed to consume fewer energy than they had been expending.

Given that the DASH food plan cuts out a variety of excessive-fats, sugary ingredients, human beings may also discover that they robotically lessen their calorie consumption and shed pounds. Other human beings may also must consciously limit their consumption.

Either manner, in case you need to shed pounds at the DASH food plan, you'll nonetheless want to head on a calorie-decreased food plan.

Other Potential Health Benefits

DASH may additionally have an effect on different regions of fitness. The food plan:

• Decreases most cancers hazard: A current overview indicated that human beings following the DASH food plan had a decrease hazard of a few cancers, such as colorectal and breast most cancers.

• Lowers metabolic syndrome hazard: Some research observe that the DASH food plan reduces your hazard of metabolic syndrome via way of means of as much as 81%.

• Lowers diabetes hazard: The food plan has been related to a decrease hazard of kind 2 diabetes. Some research show that it is able to enhance insulin resistance as well.

• Decreases coronary heart sickness hazard: In one current overview in women, following a

DASH-like food plan become related to a 20% decrease hazard of coronary heart sickness and a 29% decrease hazard of stroke.

Many of those defensive results are attributed to the food plan's excessive fruit and vegetable content. In general, consuming extra end result and greens can assist lessen hazard of sickness .

SUMMARY

DASH lowers blood stress — specifically when you have accelerated levels — and can resource weight reduction. It ought to lessen your hazard of diabetes, coronary heart sickness, metabolic syndrome and a few cancers.

Does It Work for Everyone?

While research at the DASH food plan decided that the best discounts in blood stress came about in people with the bottom salt consumption, the advantages of salt limit on fitness and lifespan aren't clear-cut.

For human beings with excessive blood stress, decreasing salt consumption drastically impacts blood stress. However, in human beings with everyday blood stress, the results of decreasing salt consumption are lots smaller.

The concept that a few human beings are salt touchy — which means that salt exerts a more have an impact on their blood stress — ought to partially give an explanation for this.

SUMMARY

If your salt consumption is excessive, reducing it is able to provide foremost fitness advantages. Comprehensive salt limit, as cautioned at the DASH food plan, may also simplest be useful for those who are salt touchy or have excessive blood stress.

Restricting Salt Too Much Is Not Good for You

Eating too little salt has been related to fitness problems, together with an multiplied hazard of coronary heart sickness, insulin resistance and fluid retention.

The low-salt model of the DASH food plan recommends that human beings consume no extra than three/four teaspoon (1,500 mg) of sodium consistent with day.

However, it's uncertain whether or not there are any advantages to decreasing salt consumption this low — even in human beings with excessive blood stress.

In truth, a current overview observed no hyperlink among salt consumption and hazard of demise from coronary heart sickness, notwithstanding the truth that reducing salt consumption triggered a modest discount in blood stress.

However, due to the fact maximum human beings consume an excessive amount of salt, reducing your salt consumption from very excessive quantities of 2–2.five teaspoons (10–12 grams) an afternoon to 1–1.25 teaspoons (five–6 grams) an afternoon can be useful.

This goal may be accomplished effortlessly via way of means of decreasing the quantity of rather processed meals on your food plan and consuming primarily complete ingredients.

SUMMARY

Although decreasing salt consumption from processed ingredients is useful for maximum human beings, consuming too little salt can also be harmful.

CHAPTER THREE

What to Eat at the Diet

The DASH food plan doesn't listing precise ingredients to consume.

Instead, it recommends precise servings of various meals groups.

The wide variety of servings you may consume relies upon on what number of energy you consume. Below is an instance of meals quantities primarily based totally on a 2,000-calorie food plan.

Whole Grains: 6–eight Servings consistent with Day

Examples of complete grains encompass complete-wheat or complete-grain breads, complete-grain breakfast cereals, brown rice, bulgur, quinoa and oatmeal.

Examples of a serving encompass:

• 1 slice of complete-grain bread

• 1 ounce (28 grams) of dry, complete-grain cereal

• half of cup (ninety five grams) of cooked rice, pasta or cereal

Vegetables: four–five Servings consistent with Day

All greens are allowed at the DASH food plan.

Examples of a serving encompass:

• 1 cup (approximately 30 grams) of uncooked, leafy inexperienced greens like spinach or kale

• half of cup (approximately forty five grams) of sliced greens — uncooked or cooked — like broccoli, carrots, squash or tomatoes

Fruits: four–five Servings consistent with Day

If you're following the DASH approach, you'll be consuming a variety of fruit. Examples of end result you may consume encompass apples, pears, peaches, berries and tropical end result like pineapple and mango.

Examples of a serving encompass:

• 1 medium apple

• 1/four cup (50 grams) of dried apricots

• half of cup (30 grams) of sparkling, frozen or canned peaches

Dairy Products: 2–three Servings consistent with Day

Dairy merchandise at the DASH food plan have to be low in fats. Examples encompass skim milk and low-fats cheese and yogurt.

Examples of a serving encompass:

• 1 cup (240 ml) of low-fats milk

• 1 cup (285 grams) of low-fats yogurt

• 1.five oz (forty five grams) of low-fats cheese

Lean Chicken, Meat and Fish: 6 or Fewer Servings consistent with Day

Choose lean cuts of meat and attempt to consume a serving of pork simplest occasionally — no extra than a few times a week.

Examples of a serving encompass:

- 1 ounce (28 grams) of cooked meat, bird or fish

- 1 egg

Nuts, Seeds and Legumes: four–five Servings consistent with Week

These encompass almonds, peanuts, hazelnuts, walnuts, sunflower seeds, flaxseeds, kidney beans, lentils and cut up peas.

Examples of a serving encompass:

- 1/three cup (50 grams) of nuts

- 2 tablespoons (forty grams) of nut butter

- 2 tablespoons (sixteen grams) of seeds

- half of cup (forty grams) of cooked legumes

Fats and Oils: 2–three Servings consistent with Day

The DASH food plan recommends vegetable oils over different oils. These encompass margarines and oils like canola, corn, olive or safflower. It additionally recommends low-fats mayonnaise and mild salad dressing.

Examples of a serving encompass:

- 1 teaspoon (four.five grams) of tender margarine

- 1 teaspoon (five ml) of vegetable oil

- 1 tablespoon (15 grams) of mayonnaise

- 2 tablespoons (30 ml) of salad dressing

Candy and Added Sugars: five or Fewer Servings consistent with Week

Added sugars are stored to a minimal at the DASH food plan, so restrict your consumption of candy, soda and desk sugar. The DASH food plan additionally restricts unrefined sugars and opportunity sugar reassets, like agave nectar.

CHAPTER FOUR

Examples of a serving encompass:

- 1 tablespoon (12.five grams) of sugar

- 1 tablespoon (20 grams) of jelly or jam

- 1 cup (240 ml) of lemonade

SUMMARY

The DASH food plan does now no longer listing precise ingredients to consume. Instead, it's a nutritional sample targeted on servings of meals groups.

Sample Menu for One Week

Here's an instance of a one-week meal plan — primarily based totally on 2,000 energy consistent with day — for the normal DASH food plan:

Monday

• Breakfast: 1 cup (ninety grams) of oatmeal with 1 cup (240 ml) of skim milk, half of cup (seventy five grams) of blueberries and half of cup (a hundred and twenty ml) of sparkling orange juice.

• Snack: 1 medium apple and 1 cup (285 grams) of low-fats yogurt.

• Lunch: Tuna and mayonnaise sandwich made with 2 slices of complete-grain bread, 1 tablespoon (15 grams) of mayonnaise, 1.five cups (113 grams) of inexperienced salad and three oz (eighty grams) of canned tuna.

• Snack: 1 medium banana.

• Dinner: three oz (eighty five grams) of lean bird breast cooked in 1 teaspoon (five ml) of vegetable oil with half of cup (seventy five grams) every of broccoli and carrots. Served with 1 cup (a hundred ninety grams) of brown rice.

Tuesday

• Breakfast: 2 slices of complete-wheat toast with 1 teaspoon (four.five grams) of margarine, 1 tablespoon (20 grams) of jelly or jam, half of cup (a hundred and twenty ml) of sparkling orange juice and 1 medium apple.

• Snack: 1 medium banana.

• Lunch: three oz (eighty five grams) of lean bird breast with 2 cups (a hundred and fifty grams) of inexperienced salad, 1.five oz (forty five grams) of low-fats cheese and 1 cup (a hundred ninety grams) of brown rice.

• Snack: half of cup (30 grams) of canned peaches and 1 cup (285 grams) of low-fats yogurt.

- Dinner: three oz (eighty five grams) of salmon cooked in 1 teaspoon (five ml) of vegetable oil with 1 cup (three hundred grams) of boiled potatoes and 1.five cups (225 grams) of boiled greens.

Wednesday

- Breakfast: 1 cup (ninety grams) of oatmeal with 1 cup (240 ml) of skim milk and half of cup (seventy five grams) of blueberries. half of cup (a hundred and twenty ml) of sparkling orange juice.

- Snack: 1 medium orange.

- Lunch: 2 slices of complete-wheat bread, three oz (eighty five grams) of lean turkey, 1.five oz (forty five grams) of low-fats cheese, half of cup (38 grams) of inexperienced salad and half of cup (38 grams) of cherry tomatoes.

• Snack: four complete-grain crackers with 1.five oz (forty five grams) of cottage cheese and half of cup (seventy five grams) of canned pineapple.

• Dinner: 6 oz (a hundred and seventy grams) of cod fillet, 1 cup (2 hundred grams) of mashed potatoes, half of cup (seventy five grams) of inexperienced peas and half of cup (seventy five grams) of broccoli.

Thursday

• Breakfast: 1 cup (ninety grams) of oatmeal with 1 cup (240 ml) of skim milk and half of cup (seventy five grams) of raspberries. half of cup (a hundred and twenty ml) of sparkling orange juice.

• Snack: 1 medium banana.

• Lunch: Salad made with four.five oz (a hundred thirty grams) of grilled tuna, 1 boiled egg, 2 cups (152 grams) of inexperienced salad, half of cup (38 grams) of cherry tomatoes and a couple of tablespoons (30 ml) of low-fats dressing.

• Snack: half of cup (30 grams) of canned pears and 1 cup (285 grams) of low-fats yogurt.

• Dinner: three oz (eighty five grams) of beef fillet with 1 cup (a hundred and fifty grams) of combined greens and 1 cup (a hundred ninety grams) of brown rice.

Friday

• Breakfast: 2 boiled eggs, 2 slices of turkey bacon with half of cup (38 grams) of cherry tomatoes, half of cup (eighty grams) of baked beans and a couple of slices of complete-wheat toast, plus half of cup (a hundred and twenty ml) of sparkling orange juice.

• Snack: 1 medium apple.

• Lunch: 2 slices of complete-wheat toast, 1 tablespoon of low-fats mayonnaise, 1.five oz (forty five grams) of low-fats cheese, half of cup (38 grams) of salad veggies and half of cup (38 grams) of cherry tomatoes.

• Snack: 1 cup of fruit salad.

• Dinner: Spaghetti and meatballs made with 1 cup (a hundred ninety grams) of spaghetti and four oz (one hundred fifteen grams) of minced turkey. half of cup (seventy five grams) of inexperienced peas at the side.

Saturday

• Breakfast: 2 slices of complete-wheat toast with 2 tablespoons (forty grams) of peanut butter, 1 medium banana, 2 tablespoons (sixteen grams) of combined seeds and half of cup (a hundred and twenty ml) of sparkling orange juice.

• Snack: 1 medium apple.

• Lunch: three oz (eighty five grams) of grilled bird, 1 cup (a hundred and fifty grams) of roasted greens and 1 cup (a hundred ninety grams) couscous.

• Snack: half of cup (30 grams) of combined berries and 1 cup (285 grams) of low-fats yogurt.

• Dinner: three oz (eighty five grams) of beef steak and 1 cup (a hundred and fifty grams) of ratatouille with 1 cup (a hundred ninety grams) of brown rice, half of cup (forty grams) of lentils and 1.five oz (forty five grams) of low-fats cheese.

• Dessert: Low-fats chocolate pudding.

Sunday

• Breakfast: 1 cup (ninety grams) of oatmeal with 1 cup (240 ml) of skim milk, half of cup (seventy five grams) of blueberries and half of cup (a hundred and twenty ml) of sparkling orange juice.

• Snack: 1 medium pear.

• Lunch: Chicken salad made with three oz (eighty five grams) of lean bird breast, 1 tablespoon of mayonnaise, 2 cups (a hundred and fifty grams) of inexperienced salad, half of cup (seventy five grams) of cherry tomatoes, half of tablespoon (four grams) of seed sand four complete-grain crackers.

• Snack: 1 banana and half of cup (70 grams) of almonds.

• Dinner: three oz of roast pork with 1 cup (a hundred and fifty grams) of boiled potatoes, half of cup (seventy five grams) of broccoli and half of cup (seventy five grams) of inexperienced peas.

SUMMARY

On the DASH food plan, you may consume a number of scrumptious, wholesome food that percent masses of greens along diverse end result and desirable protein reassets.

CHAPTER FIVE

How to Make Your Diet More DASH-Like

Because there aren't any set ingredients at the DASH food plan, you may adapt your modern food plan to the DASH recommendations via way of means of doing the following:

• Eat extra greens and end result.

• Swap subtle grains for complete grains.

• Choose fats-unfastened or low-fats dairy merchandise.

• Choose lean protein reassets like fish, chicken and beans.

• Cook with vegetable oils.

• Limit your consumption of ingredients excessive in brought sugars, like soda and candy.

• Limit your consumption of ingredients excessive in saturated fat like fatty meats, full-fats dairy and oils like coconut and palm oil.

Outside of measured sparkling fruit juice quantities, this food plan recommends you stick with low-calorie liquids like water, tea and espresso.

SUMMARY

It's feasible to align your modern food plan with the DASH food plan. Simply consume extra end result and greens, select low-fats merchandise in addition to lean proteins and restrict your consumption of processed, excessive-fats and sugary ingredients.

If you're considering attempting DASH to decrease your blood stress, you would possibly have some questions on different components of your lifestyle.

The maximum generally requested questions are addressed under.

Can I Drink Coffee at the DASH Diet?

The DASH food plan doesn't prescribe precise recommendations for espresso. However, a few human beings fear that caffeinated drinks like espresso may also growth their blood stress.

It's widely recognized that caffeine can reason a short-time period growth in blood stress.

Furthermore, this upward push is more in human beings with excessive blood stress.

However, a current overview claimed that this famous beverage doesn't growth the long-time period hazard of excessive blood stress or coronary heart sickness — although it triggered a short-time period (1–three hours) growth in blood stress.

For maximum wholesome human beings with everyday blood stress, three–four normal cups of espresso consistent with day are taken into consideration safe.

Keep in thoughts that the mild upward push in blood stress (five–10 mm Hg) because of caffeinemeans that those who have already got excessive blood stress likely want to be extra cautious with their espresso consumption.

Do I Need to Exercise at the DASH Diet?

The DASH food plan is even extra powerful at reducing blood stress whilst paired with bodily pastime.

Given the unbiased advantages of workout on fitness, this isn't always surprising.

It's advocated to do half-hour of mild pastime maximum days, and it's essential to select some thing you enjoy — this manner, you may be much more likely to hold it up.

Examples of mild pastime encompass:

• Brisk walking (15 mins consistent with mile or nine mins consistent with kilometer)

• Running (10 mins consistent with mile or 6 mins consistent with kilometer)

• Cycling (6 mins consistent with mile or four mins consistent with kilometer)

• Swimming laps (20 mins)

• Housework (60 mins)

Can I Drink Alcohol at the DASH Diet?

Drinking an excessive amount of alcohol can growth your blood stress.

In truth, often consuming extra than three liquids consistent with day has been related to an multiplied hazard of excessive blood stress and coronary heart sickness.

On the DASH food plan, you have to drink alcohol sparingly and now no longer exceed legit recommendations — 2 or fewer liquids consistent with day for guys and 1 or fewer for women.

SUMMARY

You can drink espresso and alcohol carefully at the DASH food plan. Combining the DASH food plan with workout may also make it even extra powerful.

The Bottom Line

The DASH food plan can be an clean and powerful manner to lessen blood stress.

However, hold in thoughts that reducing every day salt consumption to three/four teaspoon (1,500 mg) or much less has now no longer been related to any tough fitness advantages — together with a discounted hazard of coronary heart sickness — notwithstanding the truth that it is able to decrease blood stress.

Moreover, the DASH food plan may be very much like the usual low-fats food plan, which big managed trials have now no longer proven to lessen the hazard of demise via way of means of coronary heart sickness.

Healthy people may also have little motive to observe this food plan. Nevertheless, when you have excessive blood stress or assume you'll be touchy to salt, DASH can be a very good preference for you.

THE END

www.ingramcontent.com/pod-product-compliance
Lightning Source LLC
Chambersburg PA
CBHW070727260726
48660CB00007B/2761